Healthy Gut

Take good care of your digestive tract

By

Stella R. Thompson

MAIN THING

The information in this book is based on the author's knowledge, experience and opinions. The methods described in this book are not intended to be a definitive set of instructions. You may discover other methods and materials to accomplish the same end result. Your results may differ.

There are no representations or warranties, express or implied, about the completeness, accuracy, or reliability of the information, products, services, or related materials contained in this book. The information is provided "as is," to be used at your own risk.

All trademarks appearing in this book are the property of their respective owners.

This book may not be re-sold or given away to other people. If you like to share this book with another person, please purchase an additional copy for each person you share it with.

Chapter 1

What is stomach health and it's importance

You might have heard the term 'stomach health' and can't help thinking about what it implies - most likely a solid stomach is the only one that processes your food successfully. While this is valid, stomach health affects the strength of your whole body, with expanding proof proposing a solid stomach microbiome is significant for our psychological wellness, as well as a successful safe framework.

Our stomach separates the dinners we eat into a practical structure that can enter the circulatory system and go where it is required in the body. Tragically, things can turn out badly at a few phases in this cycle, from serious stomach-related illnesses to food prejudices creating issues with how our body removes supplements from food.

Yet, what happens when our guts become unfortunate, and how might we keep a good overall arrangement? Peruse on to find the fundamentals of good stomach health.

From the throat to the inside, stomach health covers the strength of the whole stomach-related framework - the pieces of our body answerable for separating our food into individual supplements we use to run our bodies. Each piece of the stomach has an alternate work and various settlements of microorganisms finish the work of separating the food into additional edible organizations.

Research shows that diet straightforwardly affects the number of inhabitants in these provinces, with calories high in fat or sugar empowering microbes that consume these supplements, and diets high in fiber empowering fiber-cherishing microorganisms that by and large live further along in the stomach. So recollect, when you eat you're not simply taking care of yourself, you are taking care of billions of stomach microscopic organisms as well, and your dietary decisions influence which microorganisms get along admirably and which vanish.

There is proof that these microorganisms might affect life span, as shown in the remarkable stomach microscopic organisms of individuals who live to be 100. Also, some stomach microbes could try and give competitors an edge, flourishing in their bodies and working on their exhibition.

A sound stomach speaks with the cerebrum through the brain organization and utilizing chemicals - this is the manner by which we know when we're eager and what we could fancy to eat. Everybody's stomach microbiome is exceptional, food varieties to such an extent that assisting one individual with flourishing may cause aggravation in others. The most widely recognized food bigotries are gluten, tracked down in wheat, and lactose and casein tracked down in milk. Certain individuals can process these parts without any issues and others will end up encountering extreme uneasiness and disagreeable side effects assuming they eat these food varieties.

The stomach is enormously significant for insusceptible capability, with the stomach wall giving an obstruction that, while working appropriately, forestalls infections, organisms, and 'terrible' microorganisms from entering the circulatory system. Sadly, this boundary in some cases becomes penetrable, referred to casually as a 'cracked stomach', and that implies these nasties can get through and make us debilitated. Conditions like crabby gut disorder (IBS), provocative entrail sickness (IBD), and coeliac illness can make individuals more inclined to create penetrability in the stomach wall, making them more powerless against sickness or disease entering the body along these lines.

Research shows that stomach well-being likewise affects psychological well-being. Known as the 'second mind', there's an explanation: we feel a lot of our feelings in our guts. Stomach microbes have the ability to animate our sensory system, sending messages to our minds through the vagus nerve. They can likewise deliver chemicals indistinguishable from those our own frameworks discharge, making them little pilots with an enormous effect on our bodies and dynamics given how minuscule they are. This correspondence between stomach and mind is known as the stomach cerebrum hub. Stress can likewise influence these microorganisms, as a great deal of them are chemical delicate, which might prompt an irregularity.

So how can you say whether you have a solid stomach?

Cristy Dean, dietician and stomach health expert for Fettle and Bloom, tells LiveScience a sound stomach can be estimated in various ways.

"This can be from how frequently we go to the loo to pass a stool, to the time it takes for food to travel through the body," she says. "Everyone is unique, but it is viewed as ordinary to go between three times each day and three times each week. Extremely sluggish or exceptionally quick travel time can demonstrate something isn't right with processing. Stools ought to be medium to dull brown, smooth, wiener like and be passed without torment or inordinate bulging or gas."

Chapter 2

What are the signs of bad gut health?

It is assessed that 60-70 million Americans experience the ill effects of stomach-related issues, making up 12% of ongoing methodology, so unfortunately stomach health is an exceptionally normal issue. Upsets to destroy well-being can happen for various reasons, however the fundamental signs that you could have an issue are:

. Swelling

. Diarrheas

. Blockage

. Acid reflux

. Sickness

Other, somewhat more dark side effects may not seem like they have a lot to do with stomach health, yet can really be areas of strength for me that something is off-base.

Weakness and unfortunate rest a recent report found that a lopsidedness in our stomach well-being can prompt upset rest examples and low energy.

Skin bothering - it appears to be odd that your outer invulnerable hindrance (skin) and interior insusceptible boundary (stomach) would be connected, however, research shows that skin disturbance can be a side effect of unfortunate stomach health.

Terrible breath/halitosis - it's a good idea that side effects of awful stomach well-being would influence the mouth, as this is the doorway to the gastrointestinal lot, yet you may not understand that terrible breath can really be a side effect that everything isn't well in that frame of mind of the stomach related framework.

Dignitary suggests paying special attention to changes and side effects that are unusual for you, as stomach health is extremely private. "Changes in gut propensity can be an indication that something is off-base, like expanded swelling, gas, the runs, indigestion, or waking in the night to pass a stool," she says. "Rest unsettling influences, expanded weariness, skin disturbance, food prejudices, and unexpected weight changes can be generally connected to an healthy stomach."

On the off chance that you assume you are encountering any of the side effects, it very well may merit visiting your primary care physician or a stomach health expert to examine likely causes and medicines.

Chapter 3

ways of further developing stomach health

1. Take probiotics and eat aged food sources

To help the useful microorganisms, or probiotics, in the stomach, certain individuals decide to take probiotic supplements.

These are accessible in health food stores, pharmacies, and on the web.

Some research trusted Source has proposed that taking probiotics can uphold a solid stomach microbiome and that it might forestall stomach irritation and other digestive issues.

Matured food varieties are a characteristic wellspring of probiotics.

Devouring the accompanying food varieties consistently may further develop stomach health:

. aged vegetables

. kefir

. kimchi

. fermented tea

. miso

. sauerkraut

. tempeh

2. Eat prebiotic fiber

Probiotics feed on nondigestible carbs called prebiotics. This cycle urges advantageous microscopic organisms to duplicate in the stomach.

Research from 2017Trusted Source proposed that prebiotics may assist probiotics with turning out to be more lenient to specific natural circumstances, including pH and temperature changes.

Individuals who need to upgrade their stomach health might wish to incorporate a greater amount of the accompanying prebiotic-rich food sources in their eating regimen:
. asparagus
. bananas
. chicory
. garlic
. Jerusalem artichoke
. onions
. entire grains

3. Eat less sugar and sugars

Eating a ton of sugar or counterfeit sugars might cause stomach dysbiosis, which is an irregularity of stomach microorganisms.

The creators of a 2015 study trusted Source in creatures recommended that the standard Western eating routine, which is high in sugar and fat, adversely influences the stomach microbiome. Thus, this can impact the mind and conduct.

Another creature study trusted Source detailed that the counterfeit sugar aspartame builds the quantity of a few bacterial strains that are connected with metabolic infection.

Metabolic sickness alludes to a gathering of conditions that increment the gamble of diabetes and coronary illness.

ResearchTrusted Source has likewise demonstrated that human utilization of fake sugars can adversely affect blood glucose levels because of their consequences for stomach verdure. This implies that fake sugars might increment glucose in spite of not really being sugar.

4. Lessen pressure

Overseeing pressure is significant for some parts of well-being, including stomach well-being.

Creature studiesTrusted Source has recommended that mental stressors can disturb the microorganisms in the digestion tracts, regardless of whether the pressure is just brief.

In people, an assortment of stressorsTrusted Sources can adversely influence stomach health, including:

. mental pressure

.Natural pressure, like outrageous intensity, cold, or commotion

. lack of sleep

. disturbance of the circadian cadence

Some pressure the board strategies incorporate reflection, profound breathing activities, and moderate muscle unwinding.

Practicing consistently, resting soundly, and eating a fortifying eating routine can likewise lessen feelings of anxiety.

5. Try not to take anti-microbial superfluously

In spite of the fact that it is many times important to take anti-infection agents to battle bacterial contaminations, abuse is a huge general well-being worry that can prompt anti-infection obstruction.

Antimicrobials are additionally damagingTrusted Source to the stomach microbiota and invulnerability, with some researchTrusted Sources announcing that even a half year after their utilization, the stomach actually comes up short on types of useful microscopic organisms.

As per the Centers for Disease Control and Prevention (CDC)Trusted Source, specialists in the United States recommend around 30% of anti-infection agents superfluously.

Accordingly, the CDC suggests that individuals examine antimicrobial and elective choices with their primary care physician before use.

6. Work-out routinely

Routinely practicing adds to great heart well-being and weight reduction or weight upkeep. ResearchTrusted Source has likewise proposed that it might likewise further develop stomach health, which may, thusly, assist with controlling heftiness.

Working out may increment species variety. A 2014 study by trusted Source discovered that competitors had a bigger assortment of stomach vegetation than nonathletes.

Notwithstanding, the competitors likewise ate an alternate eating regimen to the benchmark group, which could represent the distinctions in their microbiomes.

The Physical Activity Guidelines for Americans suggest that grown-ups take part in something like 150 minutes of trusted Source of moderate power practice every week, alongside muscle reinforcing exercises on at least 2 days every week.

7. Get sufficient rest

Getting sufficient great quality rest can further develop temperament, cognizance, and stomach health.

A 2014 creature study trusted Source demonstrated that unpredictable rest propensities and upset rest can have adverse results for stomach verdure, which might expand the gamble of provocative circumstances.

Lay out refreshing rest propensities by heading to sleep and getting up simultaneously every day. Grown-ups ought to get no less than 7 hours of trusted Source of rest each evening.

8. Utilize different cleaning items

Similarly, as antimicrobial can disturb the stomach microbiota, so too can sanitizer cleaning items, as per the aftereffects of one review. The 2018 researchTrusted Source examined the stomach vegetation of north than 700 newborn children ages 3-4 months.

The specialists found that the people who resided in homes where individuals involved sanitizer cleaning items week after week were two times as prone to have more significant levels of Lachnospiraceae stomach organisms, a sort related to trusted Source type 2 diabetes and heftiness.

At age 3, these babies had a higher weight file (BMI) than youngsters without openness to such elevated degrees of sanitizers.

9. Try not to smoke

Smoking influences stomach well-being as well as the strength of the heart and lungs. It likewise extraordinarily builds the gamble of malignant growth.

A 2018 review trusted Source of exploration distributed north of a 16-year time frame tracked down that smoking modifies the digestive greenery by expanding possibly harmful microorganisms and diminishing the degrees of useful ones.

These impacts might expand the gamble of gastrointestinal and foundational conditions, like provocative inside sickness (IBD).

10. Eat a vegan diet

Studies have demonstrated trusted sources a massive contrast between the stomach microbiomes of veggie lovers and those of individuals who eat meat.

A vegan diet might further develop stomach well-being because of the great degrees of prebiotic fiber it contains.

For instance, in one little study by a trusted Source, individuals with heftiness followed a severe vegan diet that killed every creature item, including meat, dairy, and eggs, for multi-month.

Toward the finish of the review, the members had lower levels of stomach aggravation because of the modified kinds of stomach microorganisms. They had additionally shed pounds.

Chapter 4

Food sources For Good Gut Health

1. Oats

What's not to cherish about oats? There are a lot of medical advantages to oats and oats overall since they are loaded with beta-glucans, a sort of solvent fiber that frames a gel-like substance that moves gradually through the intestinal system and assists with keeping energy levels stable and keeping you full.

Furthermore, this sort of fiber likewise assumes a part in settling glucose levels, which quite assumes a part in stomach health as an unfortunate or imbalanced stomach can affect blood sugars. Food varieties that are wealthy in beta-glucans can assist with controlling blood sugars and lower the gamble of insulin obstruction as well. Partake in a bowl of cereal with your number one product of the soil garnishes, mix oats into a sound smoothie or make breakfast oat biscuits.

2. Bulgar

Bulgur wheat is a well-known grain in Middle Eastern cooking and is a highly safe starch that goes about as prebiotics to advance the helpful microorganisms in the stomach microbiome, making it a food that welcomes stomachs. "Bulgar is an extraordinary option to quinoa or rice, as it really has more fiber and is lower in starches. The entire grain packs a nutty flavor and adds profundity to any grain salad or side dish," Santos says.

Adding bulgur to your number one dish is a simple method for adding fiber to your eating regimen since it doesn't take long to cook, making it a helpful and nutritious option for weeknight feasts. Attempt this delightful bulgur pilaf recipe that the entire family will appreciate.

3. Bananas

Bananas are a spending plan cordial method for supporting your stomach and are known to be one of the most mind-blowing food varieties for processing. They contain a kind of solvent fiber called insulin, a prebiotic that helps feed the great microbes in the stomach. In the event that you are managing awkward gastrointestinal side effects like obstruction or the runs, adding more bananas to your eating regimen could assist with easing these side effects by further developing stool consistency and generally entrail capability as per a meta-examination.

P.S. Try not to discard that excessively matured banana in your natural product container — save it for banana flapjacks or a yummy Chocolate Banana Cake.

4. Lentils

Lentils are a flexible food plentiful in key supplements like folate, iron, B nutrients, and stomach-supporting safe starches. What's going on with safe starches? Safe starch is a kind of carb that matures in the digestive organs and behaves like a prebiotic to take care of the great microbes in the stomach. Doing that helps support the stomach microbiome alongside different advantages like keeping you full longer, further developing gut routineness, and supporting heart health.

"Lentils are genuinely plant-based nourishment forces to be reckoned with, and offer a powerful portion of both fiber and protein," Santos says. Have a go at making a generous lentil soup or match it with rice for a supporting, solace dinner. Look at a greater amount of our #1 recipes with lentils.

5. Berries

From blueberries to raspberries and strawberries, berries are quite possibly the best organic product you can eat. One thing that these berries specifically share practically speaking is holding your stomach within proper limits. They contain sickness-battling properties like cancer prevention agents which assist with decreasing irritation in the stomach. A 2020 survey from the Journal of Food and Function found that berries have been shown to reduce side effects of stomach irritation.

Berries are additionally rich in prebiotics and are one of the greatest L-ascorbic acid food varieties which can further develop the stomach boundary, upgrade supplement assimilation, and proposition assurance from specific poisons. Begin your day with a simple berry summer smoothie or freeze them and appreciate them later as a supplement thick, sweet treat.

6. Yogurt

Yogurt is presumably the main thing that strikes a chord when you consider the best food sources for stomach health, and for good explanation. Yogurt is wealthy in probiotics, which are live microorganisms that keep the stomach microbiome cheerful and sound. Assuming you're encountering side effects like bulging, gas, stoppage, or looseness of the bowels, probiotics might assist with bringing some speedy help. In the event that you're lactose narrow-minded, a non-dairy probiotic yogurt braced with L. acidophilus and Bifidobacterium sp. could actually diminish lactose narrow-mindedness side effects.

Our specialists say that not all yogurts contain live probiotics, so you'll have to peruse the name on the yogurt and quest for the ones that contain dynamic or live societies to receive their full rewards. Choose a high-protein yogurt, with negligible added sugars and straightforward fixings.

7. Sauerkraut

Sauerkraut takes any dish to a higher level with its tart taste and crunchy surface. Use it on your sandwich, on a plate of mixed greens, or as a feature of a grain bowl. One more motivation to adore sauerkraut is the many stomach medical advantages it offers. Sauerkraut is a matured cabbage loaded with probiotics to help the stomach.

During the maturation cycle, microorganisms in the cabbage process its regular sugars and convert them into carbon dioxide and natural acids. This helps separate supplements in food, making them a lot simpler to process. If you're not into sauerkraut but rather have any desire to receive the stomach sound rewards, kimchi and miso are amazing choices as well. Figure out how to make your own sauerkraut in a container.

8. Pears

This supplement's thick natural product is high in cell reinforcements, nutrients C and K which assist with supporting resistance, heart health, and assimilation. To tick the stomach health checkbox, they contain insoluble and solvent fiber which are crucial for processing as they give mass to the stool while assisting with keeping your entrails moving routinely.

In the event that you're searching for an imaginative and straightforward method for carrying pears to your weeknight supper table, attempt this delightful Roasted Pork Chops and Pears recipe.

9. Dark Beans

Whether in a soup, as a plunge, or as a side dish, beans are one of the most outstanding stomach food varieties stacked with protein and fiber. In only one cup of cooked dark beans, you'll pack in around 15 grams of fiber. High in safe starch, dark beans behave like a prebiotic during the assimilation cycle to support the great microbes.

Not every person endures beans similarly, so in the event that they are hard for you to process have a go at splashing the beans for the time being and you could possibly endure it somewhat better. Take a stab at adding canned dark beans in a fried egg breakfast burrito for an additional protein kick.

10. Tempeh

In the event that you're searching for a tart and nutty method for bringing great microbes into your stomach, tempeh is the best approach. This matured soybean item is wealthy in plant protein, as well as the two probiotics and prebiotics that emphatically impact the stomach microbiome.

While cooking, make certain to keep the inside temperature under 115 degrees to guarantee the live societies stay in salvageable shape. Attempt these simple tempeh lettuce wraps for a fast lunch choice.

11. Ginger

Ginger has a wealth of amazing medical advantages. You may know about ginger's history for its capacity to alleviate an irritated stomach and other absorption concerns like queasiness. The root likewise invigorates the gastrointestinal system because of gingerol, a characteristic substance with mitigating and cell reinforcement properties.

There are countless ways of getting a charge out of it, yet one of our #1 choice is mitigating your stomach with a simple ginger tea. Wash, strip and cut the ginger. Add water and the ginger root to a little dish and bubble. Strain the tea into a cup and let cool for 3-5 minutes. Add your #1 sugar and appreciate it.

12. Swiss Chard

The more greens, the merrier. Salad greens like Swiss chard are really simple to cook and loaded up with fundamental supplements like nutrients A, K, and magnesium. Not just that, Swiss chard is stacked with fiber to take care of the advantageous microbes in your stomach while keeping up with solid cholesterol levels.

Dull mixed greens like Swiss chard are stacked with cancer prevention agents to battle irritation as well. This veggie is exceptionally flexible, making it ideal for different dishes from servings of mixed greens to soups, stews, or sautéed with different vegetables.

Chapter 5

How an "unhealthy" Gut Impacts Your Health, According to Experts

Having an unhealthy stomach isn't simply awkward and difficult, it can genuinely affect your general well-being in a negative manner. Awful stomach microscopic organisms can cause wretchedness, and tension and can expand the gamble of diabetes and stoutness notwithstanding other medical problems.

1 What Does it Mean to Have an Unhealthy Gut?

According to Freitas, "We as a whole have our novel individual microbiome like our fingerprints. There are a few similarities, yet our hereditary qualities and climate make up our microbiome. Its actual sure difficulties can radically adjust our microbiome briefly (for example anti-toxins), notwithstanding, the microbiome in a sound individual is extremely strong. Generally, an unhealthy stomach would be related to a low variety of stomach microbiota (a proportion of various types of microscopic organisms). Furthermore, a new report showed that Bifidobacteria are commonly present in larger numbers in solid versus sick people. Thus, a sound microbiome could eventually be a blend of variety and levels of explicit microorganisms, which likely incorporates Bifidobacteria."

2 How the Gut and Brain are Connected

Specialists call the stomach our 'second cerebrum' and justifiably. After the mind, our stomach or stomach-related framework has the biggest number of neurons in the body. Doctors hear regularly from patients that they never felt restless until they began encountering some issue with their stomach. The potential mind medical advantages of probiotics found in matured dairy food sources are beginning to be divulged as we better comprehend these stomach cerebrum associations. Since our stomach has its own sensory system, it can likewise produce a large number of the very synthetic substances or synapses that the mind creates including serotonin, which assumes a vital part in rest, craving, torment responsiveness, general prosperity, and is additionally known for balancing out our temperament and sensations of satisfaction. While the stomach-mind association has been perceived for a long time, as of late, specialists are finding the stomach microbiota can likewise affect cerebrum capability and the human way of behaving. A twofold visually impaired, controlled, equal review took a gander at the impact of utilization of probiotic yogurt on mind districts engaged with pressure and feeling. This study tracked down the utilization of a particular probiotic yogurt two times per day for a long time, in ladies, bringing about a muffled reaction from the region of the cerebrum that controls feeling and sensation, and changes in the reaction of the mind to pessimistic pictures. Research is continuous to find more about the association between your stomach and your mind, and what certain probiotics can mean for that association. The psyche stomach association and job of probiotics is one of the most thrilling areas of examination in the probiotics field today."

3 How an Unhealthy Gut Affects Your Overall Health

The stomach microbiota addresses an urgent connection point between the world in which we live, the food we eat, and our general wellbeing. The more we can find out about the human microbiome, the more we can use it to assist people with better overseeing everything from stomach-related issues to state of mind and to working on various parts of wellbeing or decreasing the gamble of fostering specific infections like stoutness and diabetes. The effect of the stomach microbiome on human wellbeing is sweeping, from advantages to our stomach-related and safe framework to assuming a critical part as the center of our brain-body association, which is the reason ventures to more readily comprehend this special environment are so significant. There are key glimpses of daylight to gainfully influence the stomach microbiome, like in a couple of long stretches of time of life, however with the more seasoned grown-up, and as a result of various difficulties, keeping a decent eating regimen and consolidating probiotics and prebiotics can likewise assist with dealing with a portion of these unsettling influences. The cutting-edge probiotics ought to be chosen for their capacity to supplement stomach microbiome lacks or unequally. (Sooner rather than later, we can imagine that every one of us will actually want to consume microbes or explicit probiotics that can assist with further developing wellbeing or distinguish risk factors for various issues at the earliest conceivable second, in this way decreasing the gamble of fostering a specific illness."

4 How an Unhealthy Gut Impacts Daily Life

An unfortunate stomach can influence your everyday existence, regularly portrayed by the presence of minor stomach-related issues," says Freitas. "Around half of the overall Western populace, much of the time encounters issues connected with stomach wellbeing like swelling, gas, thundering, and additionally uneasiness, which are all awkward and can adversely affect personal satisfaction."

Summary

Keeping a solid stomach adds to better general health and resistant capability.

By making suitable ways of life and dietary changes, individuals can modify the variety and number of microorganisms in their stomachs to improve things.

Good adaptations an individual can make incorporate taking probiotics, following a fiber-rich veggie lover diet, and keeping away from the pointless utilization of anti-microbial and sanitizers.

Another basic way of life changes an individual can incorporate getting sufficient rest and practicing routinely.

Nonetheless, an individual ought to converse with their primary care physician prior to rolling out any uncommon improvements to their eating routine. This is on the grounds that for certain individuals, for example, those with a touchy inside disorder or other ailments, probiotics and fiber-rich or vegan diets may not be useful.